Affordable Paleo Recipes

Budget-Friendly Paleo Meals You Can Take Anywhere

Here is your FREE Bonus! Just head over to Paleodebunked.com or click the image below.

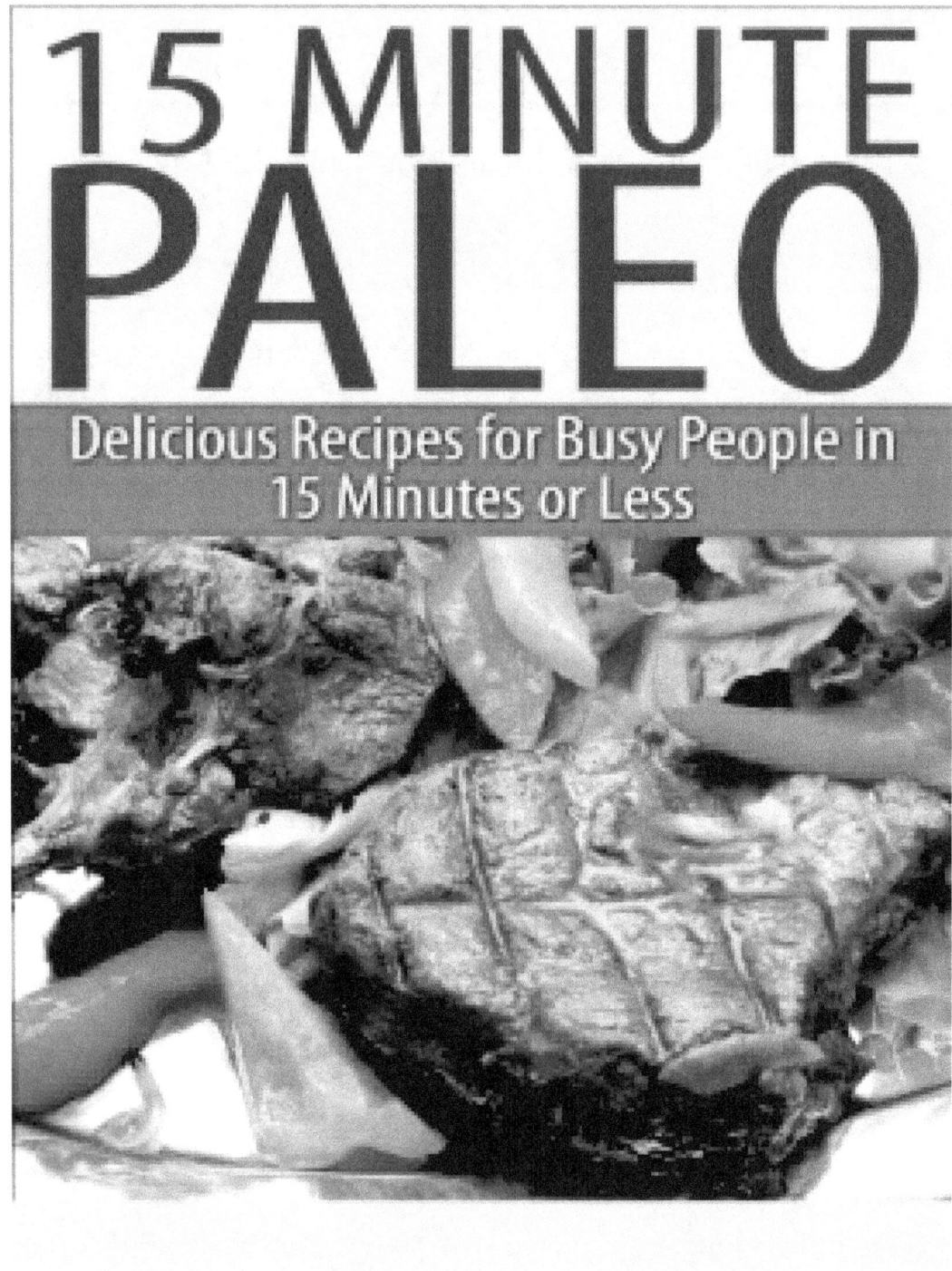

Disclaimer and Terms of Use:

Effort has been made to ensure that the information in this book is accurate and complete, however, the author and the publisher do not warrant the accuracy of the information, text and graphics contained within the book due to the rapidly changing nature of science, research, known and unknown facts and internet. The Author and the publisher do not hold any responsibility for errors, omissions or contrary interpretation of the subject matter herein. This book is presented solely for motivational and informational purposes only.

Contents

About the Book

This recipe book is for Paleo diet followers who are looking for easy-to-make and easy-to-pack foods to bring anywhere, whether it's to the office or to the gym. We've incorporated all the great Paleo diet guidelines into meals that are delicious, healthy and convenient for anyone leading a busy lifestyle. With several recipes for breakfast, lunch, dinner, snacks and dessert, you're bound to find some new Paleo favorites to whip up in your own kitchen!

Introduction

The Paleo Diet is meant to bring our eating habits in tune with our own evolution. Basically, it's all about eliminating modern processed foods and looking for ways to eat only the things our prehistoric ancestors could hunt for or find. This includes meats, fish, nuts, leafy greens and seeds.

Our genetics haven't changed much since the time of the hunter-gatherers. Those tall, muscular, athletic cavemen loaded up on meat and vegetables, and not much else. Modern men on the other hand have become dependent on grains like bread, pasta, corn and rice... and what's worse, we've become addicted to sugar as well. The Paleo Diet eliminates sugar, so unless you're getting your share of sweets from fresh fruit, you can forget about it.

The Paleo Diet focuses on various meats, fish and seafood, fresh fruits and vegetables, eggs, nuts and seeds, and healthy oils such as olive oil, flaxseed oil and coconut oil. You'll also have to steer clear of dairy, grains, legumes, starches and alcohol.
If you want to burn off stored fat, stabilize your blood sugar levels, have more balanced energy throughout the day, and prevent diseases known to be caused by consuming too much sugar such as diabetes, then the Paleo Diet is for you.

It eliminates all of these foods that are actually really low in nutrition and high in calories, while feeding your body with nutrient-dense whole foods.

The Paleo Diet helps bring you back to how human beings were made to eat. It re-educates your body to run on less processed carbs and more lean protein so that you can tap into your fat stores, lose weight, and get healthier in the process.
This book will help you whether you're just starting out on the Paleo Diet or have been following it for quite awhile. We've got simple and delicious recipes that won't break the bank. Better yet, all of these recipes are easy to pack, so you can take them anywhere!

Breakfast

Paleo Egg Muffins

Makes 6 servings.

1 lb. of bacon bits
1 dozen eggs
1/2 cup of coconut cream
1/2 tsp. salt
Black pepper to taste
1 1/2 cup grated vegan cheddar

Preheat oven to 325 F (165 C). Take a muffin tray for baking and grease it with coconut oil or olive oil. Distribute bacon bits at the bottom of the muffin compartments. Set aside.

Take big bowl and whisk cream, salt, pepper and eggs. Pour the resulting batter over your bacon bits and top with grated cheddar. Bake for 30 minutes or until the muffins are cooked through. Remove from baking tray and cool. Pack it in a brown back for a quick breakfast on the go!

Tip:
Coconut milk can be made into coconut cream. Take 1 can or 14 oz of full fat coconut milk and refrigerate for about 6-8 hours or overnight. Scrape out the cream into a bowl. The milk can be saved for later recipes or smoothie recipes. Add half a tablespoon of vanilla extract and 2 tablespoons of raw honey. Beat with a handmixer for about 10 minutes to incorporate the honey until the color is light.

Spinach Frittatas

Makes 4 servings.

1 teaspoon olive oil

1 garlic clove, minced

3 cups baby spinach leaves

3 whole eggs

4 egg whites

¾ teaspoon salt

¼ teaspoon ground black pepper

½ onion, chopped

¼ cup red bell pepper, minced

2 waxy red or white potatoes, peeled and shredded

2 tablespoons chopped fresh basil

¼ cup shredded Parmesan cheese

Preheat a broiler and position the rack 4 inches from the heat source. Heat 1/2 teaspoon of the olive oil in a large frying pan over medium heat. Sauté the garlic until softened for about 1 minute. Stir in the spinach and cook until it wilts, 1 to 2 minutes. Transfer to a bowl. Set the frying pan aside. In a bowl, whisk together the whole eggs and egg whites. Stir in 1/4 teaspoon of the salt and the pepper. Set aside.

Return the frying pan to medium heat and heat the remaining 1/2 teaspoon olive oil. Add the onion and sauté until soft and translucent, about 4 minutes. Stir in the remaining 1/2 teaspoon salt, the bell pepper and the potatoes and cook until the potatoes begin to brown but are still tender-crisp, 4 to 5 minutes.

Spread the potatoes in an even layer in the pan. Spread the spinach evenly over the potatoes. Sprinkle with the basil. Pour in the beaten eggs and sprinkle evenly with the cheese. Cook until slightly set, about 2 to 3 minutes. Carefully place the pan under the broiler and broil until the frittata is brown and puffy and completely set, about 3 minutes. Gently slide onto a warmed serving platter and cut into wedges. Enjoy.

Egg Omelets in Ham

Makes 6 servings.

12 slices of ham

1 dozen eggs

1 handful of chopped red bell peppers

1 handful of finely chopped onions

Salt and pepper to taste

Coconut oil

Preheat oven to 350 F (175 C). Take a muffin tray with at least 12 compartments and grease the muffin compartments with coconut oil or lard. Line the compartments with ham slices. Get a large bowl and whisk together eggs, peppers, onion and salt and pepper. Pour the mixture into the muffin compartments lined with ham. Bake for 15 to 20 minutes or until eggs are cooked through. Take the tray out of the oven and cool. Enjoy!

Almond Butter & Banana Breakfast Shake

Makes 1 serving.

1 cup of coconut milk

1 ripe banana

2 tbsp. almond butter

Crushed ice

Combine the milk, crushed ice, banana and almond butter in a blender. Blend until smooth. Serve chilled.

Paleo Steak and Eggs

Makes 1 serving.

1 elk round steak (or steak of your choice)

1-2 pieces of bacon

2 eggs

½ yellow onion, diced

½ teaspoon dried basil

Salt and pepper to taste

2 tsp. coconut oil

Season your steak with salt and black pepper. Heat a large skillet over medium heat. Add 1 tsp. of oil and sauté the onions. Add salt and pepper to the onions to your liking. While the onions are caramelizing, add the dried basil to your steak. Wrap the bacon around the steak and add the steak to the skillet. Cook the steak for about 3 to 4 minutes or whichever way you like it, then set it on a plate.

Get another small frying pan, add the remaining tsp. of oil, lard or tallow, and fry two eggs. Add salt and pepper as desired. Lay the fried eggs on top of the steak. If you'd like, you could add more caramelized onions and maybe a bit of avocado on top for additional healthy fats.

Scrambled Eggs and Salmon

Makes 2 servings.

1 tsp. coconut oil

4 eggs

1 tbsp. water

4 ounces of salmon bits

1/2 avocado

Black pepper to taste

4 chives, minced

Place a medium skillet over medium heat. Add oil of your choice. While the oil is heating up, crack the eggs into a small bowl. Add a bit of water and beat with an egg beater. Add the eggs to the skillet along with salmon. Stir continuously until eggs are fluffy. Remove from heat, set on a plate and top with black pepper, avocado and chives. Enjoy!

Denver Omelet

Makes 2 servings.

4 eggs

1 tsp. coconut oil or olive oil

1/2 of a large onion, diced

1 bell pepper, diced

1 large tomato, diced

1 cup spinach

1/4 lb. ham, cooked and diced

Salt and black pepper to taste

Wash and chop vegetables. Set aside. Crack eggs into a bowl and beat with an egg beater until frothy. Set aside. Heat a large skillet over medium heat. Add oil and wait until the oil is hot. Add half of the onions and bell peppers and cook, stirring until translucent. Pour the beaten eggs into the skillet. Wait for it to set, then scrape the edge off on one side and flip over so that the uncooked egg on top can spread to the skillet. Add the rest of the onions, bell peppers, tomatoes, spinach and ham to one side of the omelets and cook for a couple of minutes or until the egg is almost fully set. Use a spatula to fold the empty half of the omelet over the ham and vegetables. Cook for a minute longer then serve.

Crispy Prosciutto-Wrapped Asparagus

Makes 3 servings.

15 asparagus spears, stems trimmed 2" from the bottom

8 thin slices of prosciutto ham, cut in half lengthwise

Salt and pepper to taste

2 tbsp. coconut oil or olive oil

Balsamic vinegar

Heat up a broiler to high, with the rack arranged 5 to 6 inches from the heat source. Arrange the asparagus spears on a baking sheet and drizzle with oil, then season with salt and pepper. Make sure the spears are all evenly coated with oil and seasoning. Remember not to add too much salt, since prosciutto ham is already quite salty by itself. Wrap the strips of prosciutto in a downward spiral around the asparagus spears, starting just under the scaly tip of the vegetable towards the cut end. Place the wrapped asparagus spears back on the baking sheet and arrange them so that the spears don't touch one another (otherwise, the ham won't end up as crispy as it should be). Pop the baking sheet into the broiler and broil for 3 to 5 minutes or until the prosciutto becomes crispy and the asparagus tenderizes. You should toss the asparagus once you reach the halfway point to make sure it cooks evenly. When the asparagus is cooked, arrange it on the plate and drizzle with balsamic vinegar. Enjoy!

Lunch

Eggplant Goat Cheese Roll Ups

Makes 3 two-roll servings.

1 very large, wide eggplant

1/2 tsp. dried oregano

3 medium tomatoes, seeded and chopped

1 whole small green onion, minced

1 clove of garlic, minced

2 tbsp. vegan cheese

Olive oil

Get the eggplant and cut it lengthwise into 1/3-inch-thick slices. Discard the slices from the 2 outermost edges of the eggplant. Take the other slices and rub a dash of salt, pepper and oregano into both sides of each slice, then follow up the salt with a light brushing of olive oil. Preheat broiler. Once the broiler is hot, place the eggplant on the rack broil for 2 minutes on each side or until the eggplant turns golden brown. Combine onion, tomatoes and garlic in a bowl. Spread each slice with 1/2 tbsp. goat cheese and some of the tomato mixture, then roll up the slices beginning with the short side. Serve immediately. Enjoy!

Garlic Shrimp and Artichoke Hearts

Makes 2 servings.

1 pound of raw shrimp, peeled and deveined

2 cloves garlic, minced

1 jar (14 oz.) of canned artichoke hearts

2 tbsp. of capers

Pepper to taste

2 tbsp. coconut oil

Mince the garlic cloves and chop the artichoke hearts into small bits. Heat coconut oil in a large saucepan over medium heat. When the oil is hot, sauté the garlic cloves until they turn translucent and soft, but not brown. Add shrimp, capers and artichoke bits. Cook, stirring occasionally for about 4 minutes or until the shrimps turn pink. Season with pepper to taste. Serve and enjoy!

Baked Eggs in Bell Peppers

Makes 6 servings

3 bell peppers of varying colors

4 tbsp. almond butter

2 tbsp. coconut oil

4 cloves of garlic, diced

1 cup of chopped onions

1 lb. of squash, peeled, seeded and cut into cubes

1 tsp. dried thyme

Salt and ground pepper to taste

1 cup of vegan cheddar cheese

6 eggs

Prep a large baking tray and preheat oven to 375 F (190 C). Slice bell peppers into halves lengthwise and scoop out the insides. Arrange bell peppers, cut side up, on the tray. Roast in the oven for 15 to 20 minutes. Remove and drain any liquid from the inside of the pepper. Set peppers aside.

Heat a skillet over medium heat and add butter and coconut oil. Sauté garlic and onions, add squash, thyme and salt and cook for 5 minutes or until squash is soft. Reduce heat and top squash with cheese. Spoon some of the squash into each pepper half, leaving a hollow spot in the center for the eggs. Bake for the squash-filled peppers for 10 minutes then remove from oven. Crack an egg into each pepper being careful not to spill. Season with pepper and bake for another 10 minutes or until the eggs set.

Broccoli and Red Pepper Salad

Makes 4 servings

2 green onions, chopped

1 large red pepper, chopped

½ cup fresh parsley, chopped (optional)

⅓ c. pine nuts (toasted)

1 garlic clove, minced

2 tsp. mustard (Dijon)

1 tsp. raw honey

1 Tbsp. zest from a lemon

¼ cup juice from a lemon

5 Tbsp. coconut oil or olive oil

Salt and black pepper to taste

2 cups of broccoli or cauliflower

Steam broccoli until tender for 4 to 6 minutes. Chop. Add parsley, onions, and toasted pine nuts. Set aside. In a large bowl, whisk together oil, garlic, Dijon, raw honey and zest and a dash of salt and pinch of pepper. Add remaining ingredients and mix well. You can marinate the salad in the refrigerator for a few hours to let the flavors settle, or you can serve it at room temperature. Enjoy!

Pork Loin on Baked Sweet Potato

Makes 1 serving.

1 small sweet potato, washed and cleaned

2 cloves of garlic

180 grams (about ½ lb) pork loin

1 tsp. olive oil

3/4 tsp. crushed black pepper

1/2 tsp. salt

1 tsp. chopped rosemary

1/2 orange, cut into thin slices

Salt and pepper to taste.

Dressing:

1 tsp. white wine vinegar

1/2 orange juice and zest

1 tsp. honey

1/2 tsp. Italian seasoning or fresh chopped rosemary

2 tbsp olive oil

Preheat your oven to 350 F (175 C). Wrap the sweet potatoes along with the garlic cloves in a piece of tin foil and bake them in the oven for 20 minutes or until tender. On a small baking dish, drizzle pork loin with olive oil and season with salt, pepper and rosemary. Lay the sliced oranges on top of the pork and roast for about 30 minutes. Mix all ingredients for the dressing in a shaker. Set aside. Arrange the pork loins on top of the baked sweet potatoes and drizzle with dressing.

Pan-Seared Salmon with Caper and Lemon Vinaigrette

Makes 1 serving.

1 150-gram salmon fillet

1 tsp. capers, drained and chopped

1 tbsp. extra virgin olive oil

Salt and pepper to taste

Dressing:

2 tsps. Dijon mustard

1 lemon, zest, juice reserved

1/3 cup extra virgin olive oil

1/4 tsp. salt

A pinch of pepper

Warm 1 tbsp. olive oil over medium heat in a pan. Season the salmon filled in salt and pepper. Sear the fillet in the frying pan until each side is lightly browned. Transfer fish to a serving plate and set aside. Sauté the capers for 1 minute or until lightly crisp. Sprinkle the capers over the salmon. For the dressing:

Combine lemon juice and zest with mustard in a bowl. Pour the olive oil and mix. Drizzle a little bit on salmon or serve on the side.

Greek Salad and Chicken

Makes 4 servings.

2 1/2 tbsp. red-wine vinegar

1 tbsp. extra-virgin olive oil

½ teaspoon dried oregano

1/2 tsp. garlic powder

1/8 tsp. sea salt

1/8 tsp. freshly ground pepper

1 tbsp. lemon juice

1/4 cup or 16 pieces of Kalamata olives, sliced

½ cucumber—peeled, seeded and sliced into thick half-moons

1/4 cup cubes of almond feta cheese

1 medium tomato cut into wedges

½ green pepper (capsicum)—julienned

1/4 cup(s) finely chopped red onion

3 cups of chopped romaine lettuce

1 1/4 cup(s) (about 6 oz.) chopped cooked chicken breasts

Whisk vinegar, oil, dill or oregano, garlic powder, salt, and pepper in a large bowl. Add the rest of the salad ingredients into the bowl; toss well until the dressing is evenly distributed, then serve. Enjoy!

Paleo Taco Salad

Makes 4 servings.

1 lb. ground beef

8 tbsp. taco seasoning (see below)

Several leaves of romaine lettuce

1 cucumber

2 ripe avocados

2 medium ripe tomatoes

1 large red bell pepper

4 green onions

1 cup salsa

Taco seasoning:

8 tbsp. chili powder

8 tsp. paprika

8 tbsp. ground cumin seed

Dash of dried oregano

8 tsp. garlic powder

4 tsp. cayenne pepper

Combine all spices for taco seasoning. Mix well.

Cook ground beef in a pan over medium heat. Stir frequently. While the beef is cooking, lay lettuce leaves on 4 plates and set aside. Chop the vegetables and divide equally into 4 portions, arranging these on top of the lettuce plates. When beef is almost cooked, add 4 tbsp. of taco seasoning and mix well so that beef is evenly coated with spices. If the meat is too dry to mix well, you can add a little bit of water or oil. When meat is fully cooked, scoop it onto the vegetables in 4 equal portions. Top with salsa. Enjoy!

Dinner

Marinated Chicken Breasts

Makes 4 servings.

2 tbsp. red wine vinegar

3 tsp. dried oregano and thyme

1 tbsp. Dijon mustard

1 tbsp. honey

2 tsp. garlic or onion powder

1/4 cup extra-virgin olive oil

Salt and freshly ground black pepper to taste

2 whole boneless, skinless chicken breasts, a total of 12 oz.

(Each serving is ½ breast or about 3 oz.)

Combine the herbs, mustard, vinegar, honey, garlic or onion power and olive oil in a zip-lock bag. Seal the bag and shake it to mix up all the ingredients. Place the chicken breasts in the bag and marinate for up to 24 hours. Bake them in the oven on a cookie sheet at 375 F (190 C) for 10 minutes per side, or place the breasts on a grill and cook for about 4 minutes per side.

Caesar Salad with Shrimp

Makes 4 servings of about 2.5 cups each

½ cup Caesar salad dressing

1 tbsp. juice from a lemon

½ tsp. ground black pepper

¾ lb. raw peeled large shrimp (veins removed)

6 c. romaine lettuce (torn)

2 tomatoes, sliced

¼ c. dairy free parmesan cheese (shredded)

1 lemon sliced

Heat a grill to medium heat. Mix the salad dressing with the juice from a lemon and the ground pepper and marinate the shrimp. Grill for 3 minutes per side or until no pink remains. Toss greens, tomatoes and dressing in a large bowl. Sprinkle with grilled shrimp and parmesan cheese. Garnish with lemon wedges (optional). Enjoy!

Asparagus and Eggs

Makes 1 serving.

5-6 stalks Asparagus

1 teaspoon olive oil

¼ teaspoon salt

2 eggs

¼ cup dairy free parmesan cheese (*optional)

Pepper to top

Heat olive oil in a skillet over medium heat. Cut off ends of asparagus and add to skillet along with salt. Shake skillet to coat asparagus and cook until tender, 4-5 minutes. Spread asparagus out and crack eggs in the center. Sprinkle cheese over asparagus and eggs. Cover and let cook until egg whites are firm and yolk is done to desired consistency. Serve with freshly cracked pepper.

Grilled Chicken and Spinach Salad

Makes 4 servings.

4 boneless skinless chicken breasts (3 oz. each)

8 oz. baby spinach

Few thin slices of red onion

½ sweet red bell pepper, sliced into strips

1 ½ cups tomato halves

1 carrot, sliced into ribbons

Home-made or store-bought balsamic vinaigrette

Marinade:

2 tbsp. fresh squeezed lemon juice

1 tsp. dried oregano

1 tsp. garlic, crushed

Salt and fresh ground black pepper to taste

Combine the marinade ingredients and pour over chicken, let the breasts marinade in the refrigerator a minimum of two hours, but preferably up to 24 hrs. Preheat your grill to medium-high and lay the chicken on the grill. Cook the chicken until well browned on both sides and firm, about 4 minutes on each side. Set aside. Divide the salad ingredients onto 4 plates and top with grilled chicken, then drizzle with balsamic vinaigrette.

Avocado and Almond Salad

Makes 2 servings.

2 cups chopped romaine lettuce

1 chopped avocado

1 chopped medium tomato

1/4 cup almonds, salted and toasted

2 tbsp. diced green onion

1 tbsp. diced fresh cilantro

1 tbsp. olive oil

2 tsp. lime juice

1/4 tsp lime zest

1/4 tsp salt

1 tsp white balsamic vinegar

1/2 tsp ground black pepper

Place the drained and rinsed black beans into a bowl; add the vinegar and mix until well combined. Set aside. Place the avocado, tomato, red onion, and cilantro together in a bowl. Combine the lime juice, garlic, and oil into a small container, whisk until well combined. Pour avocado mixture in with the almonds then drizzled the top with the lime mixture. Mix until evenly coated and well combined. Season with sea salt and freshly cracked pepper, to taste. Serve immediately.

Paleo Chicken Stir Fry

Makes 4 servings.

1 tbsp. coconut oil or olive oil

2 tbsp. sesame oil

1/4 cup of tapioca flour

4 tbsp. coconut aminos

Salt and white pepper to taste

2 tsp. vinegar

1 tsp. fish sauce

2 onions, sliced

3 inches of fresh ginger root, peeled and finely chopped

6 garlic cloves, smashed and finely chopped

1/2 lb. of shiitake mushrooms, sliced

1 lb. of green cabbage, cut into small pieces

1 bunch of scallions

1 lb. of broccoli, cut into bite sized pieces

1/2 cup chicken broth

1 pound of chicken thighs, cut into bite sized cubes

Prep veggies by slicing onions and mushrooms, and chopping up the garlic, ginger and other vegetables. Cut scallions, dividing it into the light and dark parts. Smash and chop the scallion whites and slice the dark parts of the scallion into 2-inch pieces. Combine garlic, ginger and scallion whites in a small bowl. In another bowl, add 3 tbsp. of the mixture you just made to the bite-sized chicken cubes. Add 1 tbsp. of toasted sesame oil, 2 tbsp. of coconut aminos, a dash of white pepper and salt. Mix well and marinate in the refrigerator.

Chop the cabbage into 1-inch pieces. Slice shiitake mushrooms and broccoli into bite sized pieces. Combine the remaining garlic and ginger mixture with sesame oil, 2 tbsp. of coconut aminos and another dash of salt and pepper. Stir in chicken broth and mix well.

In another bowl, mix tapioca flour with 1/4 cup of cold water. Heat a large skillet over high heat and add 1/2 tbsp. of coconut oil. Sauté the sliced onions until translucent. Add cabbage. Cook for a few minutes, stirring constantly. Add broccoli and mushrooms. Cook for a couple more minutes. Remove vegetables and place in a bowl. Set aside.

Add 1/2 tbsp of coconut oil to the skillet and cook the marinated chicken thighs for about 2 minutes, untouched. Stir, then cook for 2 more minutes. Add the garlic, broth and coconut amino mixture to the chicken and bring to a boil. Cover and cook for about 3 minutes. Pour in tapioca starch and stir to thicken the sauce. Put the vegetables back in the skillet along with the scallions. Toss until everything is completely covered with sauce, then remove from heat and serve immediately. Enjoy!

Snacks and Desserts

Prosciutto-Wrapped Pears

Makes 4 servings.

3/4 cup balsamic vinegar (will be reduced to 3 tablespoons)

2 pears, each cut into 8 wedges and cored

8 thin slices (4 oz.) prosciutto ham, cut in half lengthwise

In a small saucepan, add the balsamic vinegar and place it over medium heat. Bring the vinegar to a simmer and then decrease heat to medium-low. Cook for 5-7 minutes until vinegar is a syrupy consistency. Transfer to a small bowl and set aside. The balsamic will continue to thicken as it sits. Proceed to wrap each pear wedge with slices of prosciutto and place a skewer in its center. Using a teaspoon, drop small dollops of balsamic glaze on your serving dish. Place the prosciutto skewers atop the balsamic glaze and serve.

Balsamic Baby Carrots

Makes 10 servings.

4 bunches baby carrots

50g or 1/4 cup, firmly packed coconut sugar

30g or 2 tbsp. almond butter, melted

2 tbsp. balsamic vinegar

Trim stems from the carrots. Scrub to remove any dirt. Peel. Preheat oven to 350 F (180 C). Place the carrots in a large 3L (12-cup) capacity glass or ceramic ovenproof baking dish. Combine the sugar, butter and vinegar in a small bowl. Pour over the carrots. Season with salt and pepper. Toss to coat. Bake in oven, tossing occasionally, for 45 minutes or until the carrots are tender. Arrange on a serving platter. Drizzle over the glaze to serve.

Cinnamon Oranges

Makes 4 servings.

4 navel oranges

2 tablespoons orange juice

2 tablespoons lemon juice

1 tablespoon sugar

1/4 teaspoon ground cinnamon

With a sharp knife, remove rind and white pith from oranges. Cut each into 5 or 6 slices and arrange on 4 plates. Whisk together orange juice and lemon juice, sugar and cinnamon. Spoon over the orange slices. Enjoy.

Paleo Trail Mix

Makes 7 cups.

½ cup coconut oil, melted

1 cup fresh pineapple, cut into 1-inch cubes

1/2 cup almonds, chopped

1/2 cup raw pumpkin seeds

1/2 cup raw macadamia nuts, chopped

1/2 cup pecans

½ cup raw sunflower seeds

½ cup of dates, pitted and chopped

3 cups raw coconut flakes

1 teaspoon ground cinnamon

2 tbsp. maple syrup

½ teaspoon salt

1 tablespoon vanilla extract

Heat up the oven to 325 F (165 C). Cover two sheets with parchment paper or foil and set aside. In a food processor, combine pineapple, dates, vanilla extract, and cinnamon. Process until the mixture turns to liquid. Add coconut oil and blend until smooth. In a large bowl, toss all the nuts, seeds and coconut flakes together and add salt. Mix the blended mixture into the nuts and seeds, making sure they are all evenly coated. Spread the nuts and seeds onto the baking sheet in an even single layer and bake in the oven for around 35 minutes or just until it turns a nice shade of golden brown. Watch the oven carefully to make sure you don't overcook your trail mix. Cool the mix, store in an airtight container at room temperature. Enjoy!

Grab and Go Paleo Granola

Makes 2 servings.

2 cups of assorted nuts

(Almonds, macadamia nuts, walnuts, pecans or pistachios will all do the trick)

1/4 cup honey

2 tbsp. tapioca flour

1 pinch of salt

1 tsp. ground cinnamon

1/4 cup of almond butter, cut into 1-inch cubes

Preheat oven to 350F (175 C). Take a food processor and add all the ingredients except the butter. Add 1 cube of butter at a time and pulse so that the butter mixes well with the other ingredients. Once all ingredients are thoroughly blended into a rough mixture, spoon it evenly onto a baking sheet lined with parchment paper or foil. Bake for 10 to 15 minutes or until golden brown. You can keep this treat in an airtight container for a crunchy, nutty breakfast on the go.

Chocolate and Date Bars

Makes about 12 servings.

1 cup of pitted dates

1/2 cup almonds, chopped into fine bits

1/4 cup walnuts

1/4 cup cocoa powder

Pulse the nuts in a food processor until they are ground into fine bits. Add the pitted dates and cocoa and pulse even more until everything is mixed well. The mixture should look clumpy and feel slightly dry. Spoon this mixture onto a pan and place in the refrigerator for an hour to chill. Cut into bars. Enjoy!

I Need Your Help!

Please take a minute out of your busy schedule to leave a review. Your review will let readers know what to expect and what you liked about this book. I am looking forward to reading your review. Thank you so much for your feedback!

How to Submit a Review

To submit a review:
1. Make sure you are signed in.
2. Hover over **Your Account** in the upper right hand corner.
3. Click on **Your Orders**.
4. Click on **Digital Orders**.
5. Click **Write a customer review** in the Customer Reviews section.
6. Rate the item and write your review.
7. Click **Submit**.

How to submit a review from your Kindle device

Please follow the link below for instructions.
http://www.dummies.com/how-to/content/posting-an-amazon-book-review-from-your-kindle.html